Holistic Healing Explained

Holistic Healing Definition, Elements of Holistic Healing, Principles & Methods, Treatment & Benefits, Complementary Holistic Approach and Much More!

By Frederick Earlstein

Foreword

Are you as healthy as you can be or are you facing persistent physical ailments? Has your life been filled with a struggle of mental and emotional issues? Maybe you are on a quest for happiness and it has been rather elusive. You have searched far and wide for answers, to no avail. You realize that when one area of your life is weak or suffering, your whole life is affected. For instance, it does not really matter if you are wealthy, when you have to spend so much time, energy and finances on your deteriorating health.

There are certainly no quick fixes to anything, especially to health and essential happiness, but it doesn't mean that you cannot have it! You are meant to be healthy. You are meant to live happy. You don't have to live in suffering and you certainly don't have to go around in circles, wasting precious time. There is something you can do about your health and happiness.

Life is the greatest opportunity you can ever have and you have the power to make it into a great story. As a human, you are a wonderful work of art, a being that is essential to the universe. You are more than just a body with physical functions. You are more than just your mind or your thoughts. You are greater than all your emotions combined. You cannot be defined by the number of friends you have. You cannot be limited by just your spiritual beliefs. You are much more than what you earn or how much you have in the bank. All of these aspects of your life should come together in harmony if you want to experience fullness and fulfillment—the power to bring this change is in your hands.

You can create a healthy and happy life by creating a balance in these different areas and treat them as a whole. That is the power of holistic healing: bringing health to your physical, mental, emotional and spiritual facets as well as social, environmental and financial well-being.

You will know that to be able to strengthen you spirituality by learning to listen to your soul's guidance. Being whole means experiencing fullness of life and this leads to happiness and success. It is never too late to learn how you can restore balance and move in the right direction. Welcome to the wonderful world of holistic health and healing!

Table of Contents

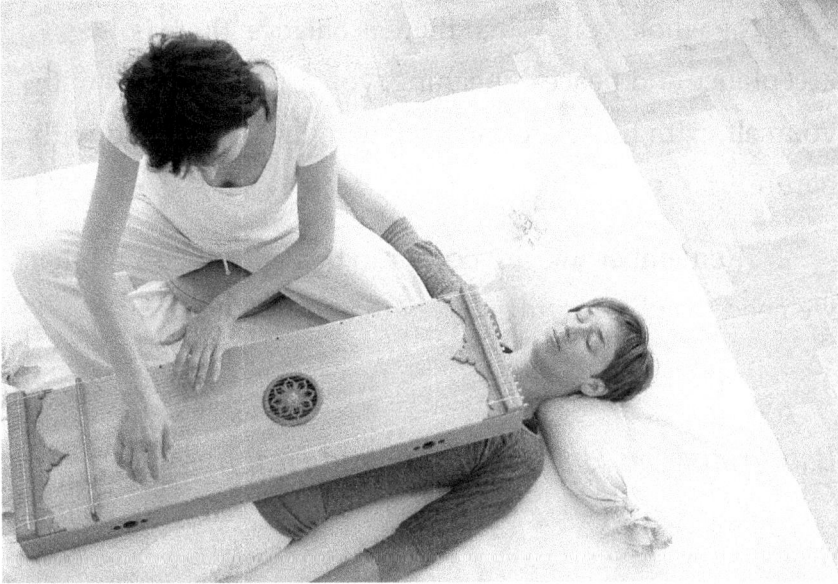

Chapter One: Holistic Health and Healing Defined

Holistic health and healing has become quite a popular approach to wellness and life in general. But holistic health and healing is not just a trend; it is an approach that considers and integrates each and every aspect of one's health, and not managing the elements individually. Holistic comes from the Greek word *holos* which means "whole". It is all about achieving and sustaining health to the *whole person.*

Understand that holistic healing is a general term that comes with wide-ranging meanings. Largely, it is the belief that you need to find balance for your spirit, mind and body as a whole instead of concentrating on the parts that are unhealthy.

While many people turn to holistic health for healing or addressing a sickness, it is best to look at it as a pathway to being whole. It is about finding and caring for your true self—the whole you. When there is balance, there is acceptance and peace—meaning, you are in harmony with yourself, with those around you, with the divine, and with nature.

Remember: we are born into this world with **all** that we need to enjoy joyful, successful and fulfilled lives.

Background on Holistic Health and Healing

Some people may think it is a new approach, but the concept of holistic healing has been in many different cultures for thousands of years. Our ancestors have been practicing and benefitting from an approach that modern health professionals ignore—treating the whole person in a natural, non-invasive and non-pharmaceutical way. Throughout history, the Chinese, Egyptians, Indians and Greeks have used holistic therapies such as massage, aromatherapy and reflexology to sustain health, prevent illnesses, and treat ailments with great amounts of success.

If you consider it, these cultures have a good number of healthy citizens compared to cultures that suffer different kinds of physical, emotional or mental ailments as they do not practice holistic approaches to health. There is truly something that is working for them that needs to be adapted. There are no boundaries to the range of illnesses and disorders that can be addressed holistically.

Today, more and more medical practitioners are utilizing holistic therapies to aid with standard medical approaches, but it is still highly likely that a medical prescription will be given first before reflexology will be advised. No matter how great the positive effects of holistic health and healing, it is only slowly taking its place in the world of health, especially in the Western culture.

One of the main characteristics of holistic healing is balancing a person's wholeness—all of his functions, his body, mind, will, emotions, spirit and relations. The practice of holistic health and healing has been applied since the 4th century BC. Socrates believed that you need to treat the body as a whole because focusing on only one part will produce bad or incomplete results. Even Hippocrates agreed that there are many factors that affect a person's health including emotional influence, nutrition, and weather, among others. Even if the word "holistic" has become part of the medical vocabulary only in the '70s, it has existed as a healing tradition dating even before ancient Greece.

Today's practice of holistic medicine is not exclusive. It can incorporate allopathic medicine in order to treat ailments and promote balanced health. There are many different holistic therapies but they all allude to the same principles that promote harmony. A popular practice in America, for instance, is the emphasis on nutrition. This is largely because modern Americans usually eat refined foods, foods that have high content of fat, sugars, cholesterol, and preservatives that often bring about various diseases. Holistic or alternative nutrition focuses on an intake of whole foods and minimizing the consumption of meat. Vegetarianism and detoxification are also a part of alternative nutrition.

Health is NOT the Absence of Sickness

People mistakenly adhere to the belief that health means the absence of sickness. While it is true that you are healthy when you do not have any disease in your body or mind, it is not the comprehensive definition of health. It is important that health is viewed in a broader spectrum. There are many factors when it comes to assessing one's wellness.

Holistic health and healing is all about knowing that the power to recover and have continuing wellness is your responsibility. It is inspiring, empowering, and overwhelming at all the same time. You have the power to choose how to be healthy and how to apply a wellness plan for your life. But before you delve into the methods of holistic healing, you need to know the elements of holistic health.

Elements of Holistic Health

There are essentially seven elements that sustain holistic health: spiritual, mental, physical, emotional, financial, social and environmental. When you understand these elements and work on balancing them in your life, then you are on the path to optimal wellness. It is imperative to note that each person is unique and the approach to achieving holistic wellness is just as distinctive. There is no single, one-size-fits-all formula to holistic health. Every person's journey is personalized depending on his or her personality, biological make-up and surroundings.

You will find information in the succeeding chapters on how you can strengthen each element in your life towards holistic wellness. Here is a general explanation of each health element:

Physical

When the physical element of health is mentioned, the first thing people often think of is exercise. While this are an important part of physical wellness, they are not the only factors that should be given attention.

Exercise entails movement but the body needs so much more than just movement. The physical body needs a healthy diet, good hygiene and adequate sleep. The best way to evaluate your physical health is to answer this checklist:

- Do you get adequate nutrition? If not, which food groups are you missing out on and which ones are in excess?

- Do you get ample, good quality sleep daily? If not, what is preventing you from getting a restful sleep on a regular basis?

- Do you practice proper hygiene? If not, what is keeping you from cleanliness and good sanitation practices?

Nutrition pays an important role in physical health. As they say, "you are what you eat." When you eat healthy foods, you are healthy. When you eat junk, then that's what you are and that's how you will feel about yourself. Nutrition is unique to everyone due of different factors such as age, gender, body chemistry, and degrees of activity. Having a balanced diet on a regular basis means that you feed your body AND your mind with good stuff. A good tip is to diversify your plate: you need a balance of food groups that will allow your body to get proper nutrients needed for energy, growth and even recovery. There are times when nutritional supplements are necessary. Some people are resolute about feeding their minds by reading books, attending seminars, and all that intellectual stuff—yet they don't pay much attention to what they eat. Remember, holistic health and healing is all about balance.

Another very important thing that can bring about good or bad effects on your overall wellness is sleep. Notice that when you get sufficient, good quality sleep, you have good control over your mental and emotional faculties. Remember, holistic healing is a positive cycle that affects all areas of your life.

Research shows that adults should get 7 to 9 hours of sleep every night. In today's busy world, it is hard for people to meet this sleep requirement. While there are many reasons as to why people lack sleep, there are simple ways that can be applied if you are adamant about bringing balance to this physical element of our health such as reducing screen time before bedtime, blocking out excessive noise and light, and having a winding down routine that can help you sleep easily and have uninterrupted rest.

Additionally, good personal hygiene is important to achieving holistic wellness. Simple washing of hands can keep germs, viruses and bacteria far from you. Brushing and flossing, bathing, trimming your nails—these may seem so trivial but including them in your daily routines build up a culture of cleanliness and wellness which helps keep you safe and healthy. When you practice proper grooming and good hygiene, you keep diseases at bay and you feel good about yourself—your confidence builds up and this is important to your mental, and even your social, health.

Mental

Mental health issues such as anxiety, depression, irritability, hyperactivity and other disorders and psychological symptoms, according to studies, are often brought about by physical illness and imbalances in the body like poor diet, lack of sleep and hormonal disparities. The brain can be affected by nutritional deficiencies, food sensitivities and allergies and other physical factors that damage the body. Mental health is likewise closely associated with emotional health. When there is an imbalance, individuals not only suffer from behavioral disorders and perception problems, they can also develop mild or severe emotional and mental health symptoms ranging from sadness, anxiety, depression, learning problems, schizophrenia, and even addiction.

In the holistic approach to health, the following are considered as factors that affect mental health:

- Inadequate nutrition (physical)

- Little to no exercise (physical)

- Hormonal imbalances (physical)

- Traumatic events, continued exposure to stress (emotional)

- Financial hardships (financial)

- Lack of friends (social)

- Destructive beliefs (spiritual)

- Blood toxicity (environmental)

To sustain mental health, you need to continually engage your mind with positive, encouraging and challenging things that will allow you to acquire new knowledge and build new skills. This practice will ensure personal advancement, growth, healthful involvement, and even promote self-discovery. You can enroll in continuing education classes; engage in debates or discussions, journal, play board games, read books, among others. Do whatever will excite you and make your mind grow. Keep the cogs in your brain working!

Emotional

How do you steer your feelings? Do you have control over your sentiments and your reactions? Can you effectively identify, evaluate, and share your feelings? Life is full of surprises—some good, some bad. It can take your emotions on a rollercoaster ride. You may have a healthy physical body, but if you cannot manage your emotions well, you can be very unstable. As you work on creating balance on this element, you can better comprehend, process, and handle how you feel and experience life. There are many ways to create balance and fortify your emotions such as journaling, meditation, stress management techniques and having a strong support group which can help you a lot when the going really gets tough.

Taking care of your physical health is an important factor as different bodily imbalances can trigger negative emotions. Conversely, emotional health can affect physical health—as well as mental health. Sustaining emotional health will allow you to be happy and productive and help you reach your full potential.

Financial

Often, a person's physical, emotional and mental health can be affected when he is facing a financial difficulty. This is why financial or economic health is an important element of holistic health, wellness and healing. To avoid financial stress, one should be mindful of sustaining a holistic approach to managing finances. This will include budgeting or addressing how you spend money, as well as managing savings, investments, and debt. It also includes understanding benefits, insurance, estate planning, taxes and other aspects of your finances. When you have a holistic approach to this element, you will reduce stress levels and how it will impact your life, personally and professionally.

Taking care of your financial health is not as exciting as making sure your body and mind is healthy. Nevertheless, it will strengthen the other health elements and you should take control of it the best way that you can.

You don't have to be a stickler, but here are some small steps you can take to help you be financially healthy:

- Pay your debts off; prioritize this as much as you can.

- Make a budget and stick to it.

- While it is good to save and invest, you can also set aside some money to reward yourself in terms of recreation, dining out and entertainment.

Social

Social health is all about connections. People are not meant to live alone. They are meant to develop positive relationships that will enhance their lives. Relationships bring out the best, and sometimes the worst, in people. But it is through these connections that people learn how to live with others and deal with conflict in an appropriate manner when they arise.

To sustain social health does not simply mean having friends—especially not having friends on social media. It is all about having a good support system, personal face-to-face relationships, that can help you go through life especially when there is struggle. Relationships with spouses, parents, children, friends, colleagues — these all matter when it comes to satisfaction and happiness. The more time you spend with others, the greater the pleasure and fulfillment you will have.

You can never understate the importance of having people around you, surrounding you with love and support. Often, when life gets tough or too stressful, and you don't have people around you to encourage you or simply be there for you, you also lose physical, mental and emotional health. As with all other elements, sustaining social health is important and interconnected with the others in your journey to holistic health and healing. Nurturing your social health will require time and effort on your part but remember that it is worth all the energy you will put into it. You will reap the benefits of establishing and keeping positive relationships in your life. Take the bold step and meet new people, connect with loved ones, and strengthen friendships. On the other hand, you also need to identify and let go of negative influences and relationships that suck the life out of you. Don't be afraid to make the right choice.

Environmental

Have you ever thought of how your personal surroundings and your community affect your health? There is a significant relationship between a person's holistic health and the environment he thrives in and it is reciprocal. This means that your environment can support your health and safety and you can support it back.

When you care for your natural environment, then it can support your everyday life in a way that is productive. For instance, when you keep your workspace uncluttered, you will be more creative, fruitful and less stressed. In your neighborhood, you can help out by joining environmental efforts such as recycling, segregation, and clean-up endeavors. You can prevent noise pollution. Living in a clean and quiet neighborhood will do wonders to your personal health. You can even practice organic farming; an eco-friendly approach where in the use of chemicals is barred and gets a healthy harvest that is not only good for your body but also for the environment. You've probably been hearing so much about caring for the Earth — then do your part. Everyone doing a small thing can cause a big, positive impact on the planet we live in. And it goes without saying that when you live in a safe, unpolluted environment, it will have a positive impact on all aspects of your health.

Spiritual

It is said that "you are a spirit, you have a soul and you live in a body." One of the most important elements of your life is your spiritual well-being. If you have destructive beliefs, chances are great that your life is heading for ruin. Your physical, emotional, mental, financial, social and environmental health is all compromised.

Spiritual health is commonly overlooked but is a very important aspect of holistic health and healing. When someone feels lost and imbalanced spiritually, there is a discontent with life and disconnect with oneself—this can lead to being emotionally unstable, loss of social interactions and relationships, lack of control over finances, emotional issues, and eventually physical deterioration. Alternatively, when someone is spiritually balanced, he or she feels fulfilled and strong. Being spiritually connected brings about a sense of completion and happiness, which positively affects one's physical, emotional and mental health and in turn brings constructive change to social, environmental and financial endeavors. This is why you should nourish your spiritual self just as you would nourish your physical body and your mind—it is carried over to other health elements in your life.

The spiritual element is unique to individuals. There will be people whose spiritual health plays a stronger role in their holistic wellness compared to others. It all depends on how people allow their spiritual health to define their lives. It is all about a sense of meaning in life, of purpose and values. Spiritual health can be nurtured through prayer, meditation, practicing mindfulness, and other relevant activities as applicable to one's belief system, philosophies or religion. The important thing is to remember that spiritual health is a personal journey. How you go about your spiritual journey is up to you, as long as you remember to strengthen it daily by making it a priority and dedicating uninterrupted time for spiritual activities. Learn to say "yes" to the important things and "no" to things that are not congruent to what you believe in.

Strengthen All the Elements for Holistic Health

In order for you to build holistic health and wellness, you need to understand these two things:

1. Wellness is unique to every individual.

2. Being healthy allows you to achieve your personal life goals.

Understand that you cannot do what another person is doing just because it works for him. The holistic approach to health is individualized. You need to reflect on each of the seven elements of health and determine which of these needs your attention the most. Prioritize this and work on it, then the rest will follow, like a beautiful cycle of positive results. As you build up and strengthen one element, you are creating a strong foundation for health, wellness and healing.

When you take your body, mind and soul as a whole and care for it in that manner, then you will be healthier and happier, and you will have the strength and passion to pursue your goals in life.

Chapter Two: Principles of Holistic Healing

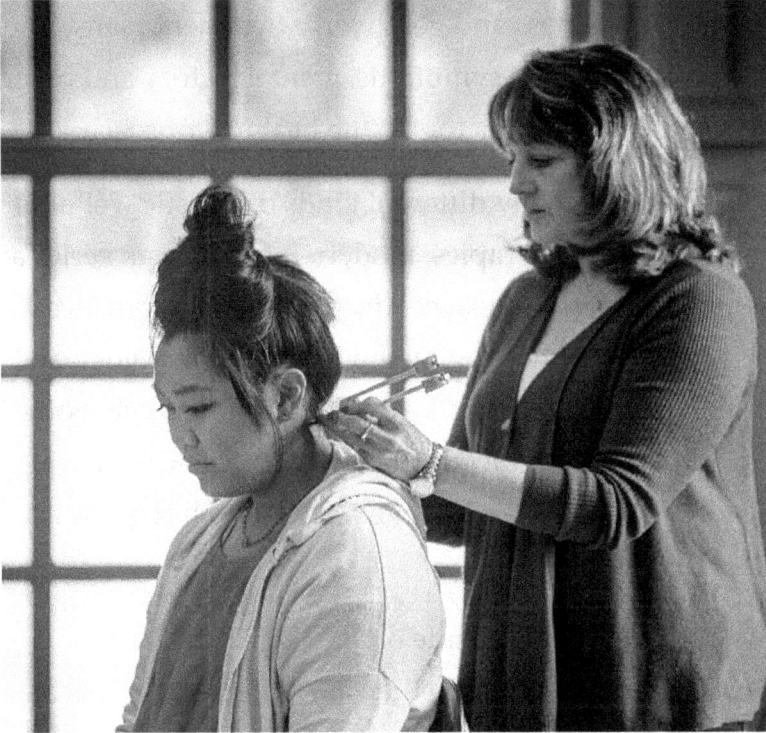

The ultimate goal of holistic healing is to restore your health holistically. This means you will strive to bring balance back into your life so that your true self can live fully. Over time, using holistic healing methods, you will be able to discard physical, mental, emotional and social toxins that are affecting you negatively. You will be able to replenish and nourish yourself with the essential healthy and positive things you need in the present and for your future.

Again, it is important to reiterate that there is no one-size-fits-all approach to holistic healing. Two individuals can have the same illness and get diverse treatment plans. Their stress levels, lifestyle, symptoms, mental history and other determinants are key factors to the healing approach.

There are many different kinds of holistic wellness plans: alternative therapies, modern medicine, surgeries and other medical techniques may be coupled with practices such as emotional healing methods, meditation, yoga and nutrition plans in order to have a holistic approach. Some people can achieve quick results while others can take a longer time before they even get a positive shift. It varies for everyone.

When individuals decide on the holistic healing approach, it can be because they are suffering a physical ailment or they have mental issues. They can be searching for ways to naturally cure their conditions. They may be disillusioned with the present techniques being used on them medically. Whatever the reason, it is important to keep these principles in mind when a holistic approach is being considered:

1. *The patient is a person, not an illness.*

This is the most important principle of holistic healing—treating the patient as a whole person. The Academy of Integrative Health and Medicine notes that holistic healing should comprise of safe and proper methods of diagnosing and treating patients to include the comprehensive study of all areas—physical, emotional, mental, spiritual, environmental, financial and social elements. While yes, there is an imbalance, the patient is not a specimen to be studied, nor a symptom to be addressed. He or she should be educated and encouraged to participate in the healing process.

2. *The chief goal is optimal health.*

Holistic healing is not just about treating the symptoms but achieving long-term health. The approach aims to achieve and sustain the perfect balance of all the elements of health. Even as it can incorporate mainstream treatments, holistic healing emphasizes natural healing so prescription drugs and surgery is not the first line of defense.

3. *The cause should be addressed.*

Holistic healing is not about treating the symptoms but attacking the root cause and cutting it off. Often, the main cause of the sickness or condition is not easily recognizable. For instance, a person suffering from a heart disease may think that it is because of his poor diet or because he does not exercise enough. But when studied closely, the heart disease can be caused by bitterness that causes toxicity to the body and damages the blood vessels. Brokenness can cause physical manifestations. If the root cause is not addressed, treating the symptoms will be superficial.

4. *The whole person must be nurtured.*

You are not just the um of your parts. You are made up of complexly connected cells, processes and systems. It is important that the whole person be taken care of and not just the parts that are ill-eased. Like the example of a person holding bitterness (emotional), the other parts (physical, mental, social, etc.) are also affected and stressed. When the whole person is nurtured and restored to recovery, the other parts will follow suit.

As much as you have the time, it is important to explore different natural options that will help you in your healing process towards mental and physical health before you turn to invasive procedures such as surgery or unnatural medicine. As you let your whole person be nurtured naturally, unhealthy parts will recover as the whole person is restored. Needless to say, when you have a medical emergency, you should immediately go to the hospital.

5. *There is healing power in love.*

Holistic practitioners believe that the approach is never without love and care. By treating the patients with kindness and gentleness, holistic practitioners are generating a powerful force that helps bring balance

6. *Prevention is as important as holistic treatment.*

A principle of holistic healing is the focus on deterrence. Like the old adage prevention is better than cure, the holistic approach works on making your "whole self" healthy so that treatment won't have to be necessary. Sickness and diseases thrive on unhealthy bodies and minds. These can be prevented.

7. *People have an innate healing power.*

The body is made to heal itself and to protect itself from diseases. When patients are encouraged to sustain optimal health through holistic approach, their minds are empowered to produce a positive effect on their physical bodies. While every case varies and every patient is distinctive, holistic health focuses on this uniqueness and not on the specific illness alone. When there is a focus on empowerment and relationships, the values are imputed on the healing process and promote the individual's autonomy over their condition. They do not become the problem, but the solution instead. Therein lies the power of holistic healing.

8. *Understand that there are both allophatic and natural alternatives that are applicable to every condition.*

Holistic healing focuses on restoring the whole person, but it is wrong to think that holism only uses the natural approach. Both allopath and natural remedies or methods, when suitably applied, can have amazing positive effects. The key is to understand that each person is unique and will require unique forms of treatments exclusive to their overall make-up.

The integration of different healing approaches is necessary as the holistic approach focuses on having all options available to a patient. Holistic health is all about giving your body the chance to do and become what it is intended to—that is to heal itself on its own. The body is wonderful and powerful and when it is in a balanced state, everything else connected with its humanity—mind, will, emotions, spirituality, relationships—will thrive. It is imperative to provide the body what it needs. Likewise, removing anything that causes it harm will aid in restoring and sustaining balance.

Take for instance medical conditions that come because of certain lifestyles—having a poor diet, sedentary living, stress-filled environments and others of similar nature can bring sickness and disease. When bad habits and lifestyles are corrected, you will see significant improvement in one's health. There are conditions where intervention of medical technology is needed, and it is not bad. You just need to complement the intervention with appropriate lifestyle change to ensure that the whole is being restored, and that is here real healing come. Sometimes, spiritual wellness and energy healing practices are necessary. Again, it depends on the person's unique needs and current health level. Not addressing the whole person is equivalent to just masking the symptoms or suppressing the real problem.

9. *Holistic healing is a lifelong learning.*

This principles applies to holistic health practitioners and patients. There is no single cookie-cutter approach, needs are always evolving and conditions are always unique. The central value of focusing on the whole person will cause both patient and practitioner to continually learn and improve on holistic health to achieve and sustain balance.

Why Choose Holistic Health and Healing

Since there is an abundance of medicines and medical methods available, why should one consider the holistic approach? Simple: because there is more to a person than just a physical body. People are highly sentient beings that live in diverse environments and experience multifaceted social structures. When you take on a holistic approach to health and healing, you are undertaking all the planes of existence. It is more than behavioral health, or mind-body medication. Holistic medicine is non-invasive, non-pharmaceutical and certainly non-traditional. Various holistic approaches include naturopathy, nutritional testing and adjustments, supplements, homeopathy, and use of essential oils, to name some. These address the different elements of health.

There are so many benefits of holistic healing to all areas of life and you will read about that in detail in a separate chapter. To put it in one thought, the all-encompassing advantage of holistic healing is this: having an intensely positive change in your lifestyle that spills over to all realms of your life.

Holistic Healing as a Lifestyle

When you choose holistic health and healing, it does not start and stop in a practitioner's office. It is all about empowering you to take control of your life. Remember that what you do on a daily basis will either nurture or damage your body, mind and spirit. Regardless of the treatment or approaches you undergo, you will not achieve balance and healing when it does not spill over to your everyday life.

The American Holistic Health Association states that the practice of holistic medicine is designed to help patients realize that they have the responsibility to manage their health. Patients are inspired and invested in cost-effective treatments that will help cure and prevent chronic illnesses and allow them to gain and sustain optimal health. As you practice holistic healing, you don't have to rely on prescription drugs or invasive procedures like surgeries in order to be well. The power to live whole and balanced, every single day, is in your hands.

Holistic healing is all about securing your health for the future, using the present time wisely and investing on balance and preventing diseases. It is a fortunate time to live in when the idea of health and wellness has become a mainstream concern. It is easy to control your lifestyle and your future. It is never too late to create that change and live life to the fullest. It is up to you to learn and apply modifications for health, happiness and a better life. You can start today!

Chapter Three: A Simple Guide to Holistic Health and Healing

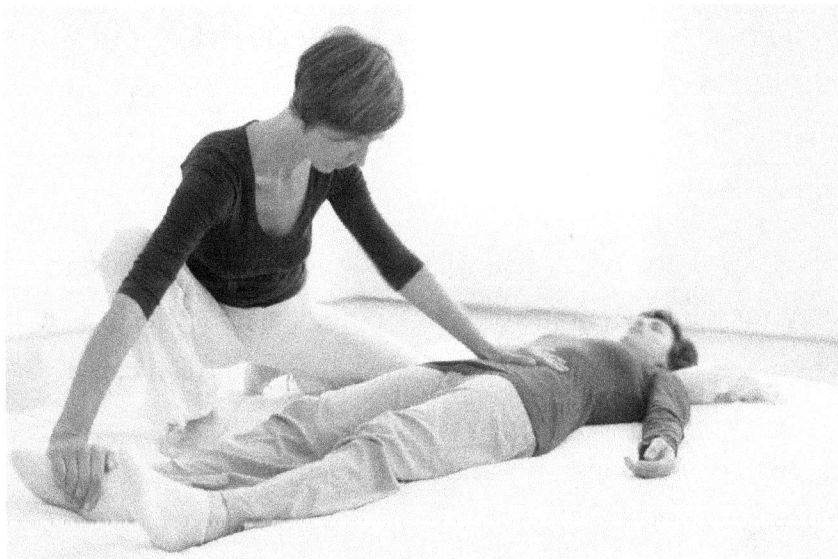

It is time to be responsible and accountable for our own lives! The main concept of holistic health and healing is to restore your balance: mind, body and emotions. As you modify one part of your whole being, you will effect change in other areas of your life to enhance your overall wellness and your outlook in life. You can cause a shift in your life and make it turn for the better. One step in the right direction, no matter how small, no matter how slowly you take it in different areas of your life, will cause movement towards becoming balanced. Holistic healing is a positive circular process wherein one good thing will lead to another good thing.

Chapter Three: A Simple Guide to Holistic Health and Healing

Wellness habits are essential in order to stay healthy and balanced. If you are healthy now and not suffering from any illness, it doesn't meant that you don't have work to do. You need to sustain that balance. If you are sick and in need of attention, then you can apply what you will learn in this chapter to promote healing, alongside appropriate implementing holistic therapies.

This chapter is a simple guide on how you can start on your journey and incorporate holistic health practices in your everyday life. Try each then choose what you can do on a daily basis. Make sure to consider that each one is important. The journey to holistic health and healing is a great adventure.

Foster a Wellness Mindset

What you think and believe in is important—it can dictate your actions and your directions. So here is what you should do: understand that YOUR health is YOUR responsibility. While doctors and holistic practitioners can and will help you, you are ultimately in charge.

The sad fact is that people don't give full attention to their health until they become sick. Remember what is always taught in school that health is wealth? It is true. When you are healthy, you don't have to spend for medication, doctor's consultations, therapies and the likes. That is the equivalent of savings! Moreover, it is far easier and better to stay healthy than to treat an illness. You don't have to settle for pain, fatigue, or anxiety. You can have a quality life now and in time to come when you make holistic health a priority. Here is how you can cultivate a holistic health mindset:

Take baby steps.

Great things start from small beginnings. Small things can add up to bring you great benefits. You don't have to take radical actions unless you are very sick and you need a complete wellness overhaul. Think of a crash diet—it doesn't bring real change to improve your health at all.

Continuous improvement will cause you to sustain holistic health. Implementing small, imperceptible yet positive changes in your life won't require too much discipline but can effectively improve your lifestyle. For example, ensuring you get to sleep 7 to 8 hours a day and cutting back on your sugar intake in small amounts every day. These will add up and you won't even notice that you are healthier and more disciplined when it comes to your health.

Nurture your spirit and soul.

Your spirit and soul are very powerful. What you believe as well as how you perceive and accept things will determine how you handle things that happen to you and around you. How do you nurture your spirit and soul? Live, laugh, love! It is more than just a nice wall décor. Learn to live life with meaning and purpose. Love yourself, love other people. Laugh often and allow your inner child to come out. Learn to connect with the divine. Practice mindfulness and being present wherever you are. These little things can make a big difference.

Keep your mind healthy and alert.

Mental well-being is often overlooked as people tend to just focus on physical needs. However, people who are mentally stressed will manifest the effects of stress in different illnesses. Some ways you can stimulate your mind include reading good books, having good conversations, improving your diet, exercising, and avoiding tobacco and alcohol.

Minimize stress.

Modern society dictates we live in a constant state of emotional and mental stress that can manifest as physical stress as well. It has become the norm that you don't even realize it when you are stressed. Depression, premature aging and various illnesses can occur and disrupt your life. Make sure that you do not put yourself in stressful situations and if you do find yourself in one, learn meditation; breathing exercises and other stress management techniques you can apply in order to minimize the effects of stress. A calm mind is a peaceful and healthy one.

Watch Your Physical Health

With a healthy mindset, it will be fairly easy to improve your physical health. Just as you minimize stress levels that affect you mentally and emotionally, you can also reduce stress on your body.

Detoxify.

Let's face it; the world we live in is polluted. There are toxins in what you eat, what you drink and in the air you breathe in. Inner toxins are also created when you worry and fill your mind with negativity. While the body is strong and can handle toxins, it can only take so much. You need to help it detoxify. Get a vegetable or fruit detox plan and follow it so you can have internal cleansing. Avoid EMF waves, personal products and other household chemicals that hinder the body's natural detox process. When you do so, you also detoxify your home and your environment. While it is not possible to take out 100% of toxins from your life, you can prevent exposing yourself to them. For instance, toxic thoughts abound in social media. Give yourself a break and cut off from being online to detoxify your mind.

Move.

Do not be sedentary — it causes a myriad of physical, mental and emotional ailments and can even cut your life short. It's not just about exercising or going to the gym. Stand up, walk, dance, jog, stretch — do anything, just don't sit for long periods of tie. Make sure to take breaks and stand up, setting an alarm reminder when necessary.

Breathe.

Learn to take deep breaths. This will help oxygenate your blood and allow you to alleviate stress. Through your nose, take in a slow, mild and deep breath and fill your abdomen.

Then release it slowly through your mouth. If you are feeling a bit stressed, take that deep breath and when you exhale, let out an "aahh" with a drop of your shoulders. To practice deep breathing, lie down and put your hands on your abdomen and take in some air without lifting your shoulders. Think of deep breathing as a detox, inhaling fresh oxygen and exhaling stale air.

Practice Prevention

Healthy habits are important, and preventive measures are equally so. As the saying goes, "an ounce of prevention is just as valuable as a pound of cure." You may not think about it while you are young and you may be prone to make poor choices and not mind them—but take heed, the effects will catch up to you in time. Avoid the damage early in life so you don't have to deal with diseases or even early death. Here are some common risky behaviors people engage in that you should avoid:

- binge eating

- binge drinking

- alcohol abuse

- drug abuse

- smoking

- unprotected sex

- drinking and driving

- talking on the phone while driving

It is not always easy to address these behaviors and you may have to get professional help, but make sure you do so. It can save your life.

Practice Healthy Habits

Here is a checklist of healthy habits you can practice:

- Eat healthy, whole foods so that you will provide sufficient nourishment to your cells.

- Hydrate well.

  - Get enough natural sunshine so that your body can produce Vitamin D needed for brain chemicals.

  - Get adequate fresh air.

  - Have ample sleep and rest every day.

- Exercise regularly—this will help your body be more flexible and strong, give you energy and promote blood circulation.

- Keep a healthy weight. Being overweight and obese can cause hormonal imbalance.

- Forgive and don't hold grudges.

- Meditate and spend some alone time every day.

- Clean your surroundings.

- Spend quality time with family and friends.

These are simple ways you can bring change to your life. However, if you are suffering from an illness and want to use holistic healing approaches, then read on the next chapters. You will discover the many benefits of holistic healing, different methods of holistic healing, how to choose the best holistic practitioner and plan for your condition and how you can take responsibility for your life.

Chapter Four: Benefits of Holistic Healing

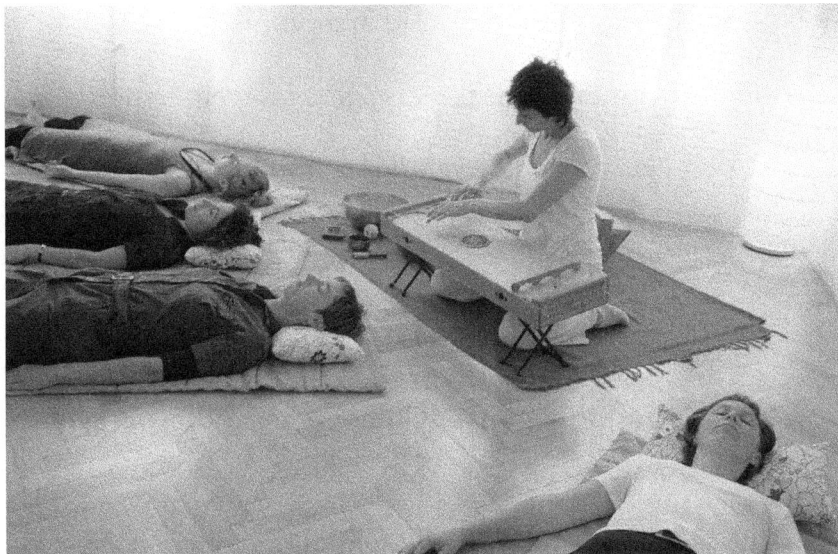

For many years in the past, the holistic approach has been shunned by medical practitioners. They considered the holistic approach as unproven and can only be applied as alternative medicine to cases that are hopeless. Fortunately, the times have changed and holistic medicine is fast becoming a standard practice. Scientific medicine and methods go together with holism, each is not exclusive. Again, holistic healing is directed at identifying the root problem or problems that causes the imbalance. It can be physical pain, poor nutrition, lack of sleep, stress and the likes. When a patient feels that what he is going through is completely considered, more than just the symptoms, he will sense love and care which proves to have a positive effect on holistic health.

Some popular benefits of holistic healing include:

- Quick relief from pain and symptoms

- Improvement of health and general well-being

- A better understanding of maintaining a balanced lifestyle

- Using more natural resources such as herbs, essential oils and natural medicine

- Being mindful of maintaining a safe and healthy environment

- Recognition and management of emotions

- Regular application of holistic methods to address sickness such as detoxification, proper exercise, modifying diets, getting ample sleep, practicing meditation and similar methods.

All these benefits will cause a patient to be on the road to recovery and empower him to maintain a lifestyle that will sustain balance.

Common Holistic Treatments and Benefits

A holistic health practitioner will guide the patient in holistic healing processes to address imbalance. Before a specific treatment is applied, a good holistic practitioner will hear one's personal story first in order to determine the best form of treatment.

The common holistic treatments include massage, fitness, yoga, acupuncture, herbal remedies, spiritual healing, mindfulness meditation and nutrition. Each of these services can have a unique positive effect on a patient's recovery and can be used individually or in combination.

Here are some holistic treatments and their benefits to patients:

1. *Acupuncture*

This old-fashioned Asian practice involves the insertion of fine needles on "acupoints". It is believed that acupuncture opens the channels of energy in one's body as it is simulated by these insertions on the skin surface. Acupuncture is not just a single insertion of a needle, but a series of procedures that help invigorate specific "acupoints" and restore the blood flow and flow of energy life force — this in turn quickens healing and helps restore balance. There are no known side effects to acupuncture and it is a generally safe procedure when performed by skilled acupuncturists. Despite skepticism and some controversy, acupuncture has gained popularity over time because of its efficacy, especially in cases of depression and chronic pain.

Acupuncture has been known to:

- relieve pain

- improve moods

- enhance healing abilities

2. Nutrition therapy

When you understand that the body is designed in such a way that it can heal itself, you will provide it with everything it needs. Nutrition response testing or NRT is a holistic technique that focuses on providing adequate nutrition in order to maintain fitness. A holistic practitioner will help you identify your nutritional needs according to your unique genetic make-up and utilize non-invasive, scientific and accurate techniques to put you on a journey towards optimal health. As with biological factors, each person has unique lifestyles, personal preferences and sensitivities to food so these factors are taken into consideration in planning the perfect nutritional diet.

Modern life can be busy and stressful, but it doesn't mean that you should neglect taking care of your body. When you are not careful, everyday life can cause imbalances. But you can recover from these as you pursue a healthy diet and a fitness lifestyle wherein you get ample hydration, good restorative sleep, relaxation, detoxification, supplementation and enough exercise. You can enjoy improved lifestyle habits, have better moods, and enhanced immune system, among many other benefits. Your body is amazing and you are meant to live life to the fullest!

3. *Yoga*

Yoga is the age-old practice of bonding the soul, body and mind in the course of different physical poses. Yoga blends meditation with various breathing techniques. The unhurried, low-impact movements are intended to extend the body and at the same time calm the mind.

When used as a holistic therapy, yoga and meditation can bring about the following benefits:

- relaxed mind

- body is stretched and tension is reduced

- awareness of body and mind is achieved

- improved sleep and moods

Yoga is a soothing way to discharge negative emotions and thoughts that are inside you but you can't seem to express. It is a great way to achieve emotional balance and control your emotions and thoughts. Yoga also helps enhance your self-confidence. So what are you waiting for? Strike a pose and let your mind get in a state of relaxation.

4. *Spiritual healing therapy*

This is all about healing the soul. It is largely believed that the soul can invoke self-healing hence it is necessary to address emotional blockages and other issues that hinder the powerful force of the soul to cause balance to the body. Benefits of this treatment include:

- awareness of self

- good management of emotions and stress

- sense of freedom

- building of confidence

- having peace

Spiritual therapy can help you learn to calm your mind and connect with your soul. This holistic healing will allow you to discover or re-discover your purpose in life and your beliefs. Not only can you relax and minimize stress, connecting with your spiritual center will allow you to live out your core values and be more self-confident.

5. *Meditation and relaxation*

Learning to quiet the mind has amazing benefits. Meditation has been used for ages to promote holistic health and healing. It has been proven to provide corporeal positive effects on one's body and mind and improves healing processes. Meditation allows a person to transcend the physical, mental and emotional stressors that affect him and enables him to find his center that causes balance. As with spiritual healing and yoga, meditation can bring about the following benefits:

- peace of mind

- healthy emotions

- good sleep

- balance of mind and body

- self-awareness and confidence

Many other holistic healing therapies and techniques will be discussed in detail throughout this book. The point of this chapter is that you cannot discount the many amazing benefits of holistic healing. When the whole person is given attention, the healing and restoration of the parts will naturally follow. Understand that holistic healing is not just a buzzword. Now that you have an idea of the benefits of holistic healing, you will grasp its importance to modern society.

Holistic Healing in Modern Times

In a world where people are faced with issues of racism, materialism, bullying, poverty, social pressures and more, the need for a holistic perspective is very vital. People go through life without a sense of purpose; they need to belong, they need direction and validation. When these issues are not addressed, mental, emotional and physical illnesses arise. When holistic connections are maintained, balanced health is achieved. Hence, getting holistic healing cannot be ignored.

There is an ongoing movement across cultures on practicing holistic lifestyles. You can see them in small relationships, communities, and commercial health establishments. More and more people are recognizing the need for the holistic approach – whether for preventing illnesses or healing. Practices include sourcing whole, locally produced foods, using natural medicines, having healthy eating and sleeping habits, doing stress-relief exercises, experiencing nature, turning to spiritual healings, going through emotional reflections and the likes. In a good way, the holistic lifestyle is helping humans be humans again.

Not only does the holistic approach benefit people suffering from diseases through experiencing lesser pain, improved health and attaining total healing, holistic healing therapies have also been known to aid in rehabilitation of addictions such as drug and alcohol. Recreational therapies, use of natural medicine, proper exercises that relieve stressors, proper nutrition, meditation and spiritual counseling have helped addicts recover and move on to full health. On another note, some pet owners have also turned to holistic approaches to take care of their beloved pets and keep them strong, happy and healthy. Methods include proper nutrition, natural supplements, good exercise, massage, and natural therapies like acupuncture instead of invasive medicines.

Chapter Five: Methods of Holistic Healing

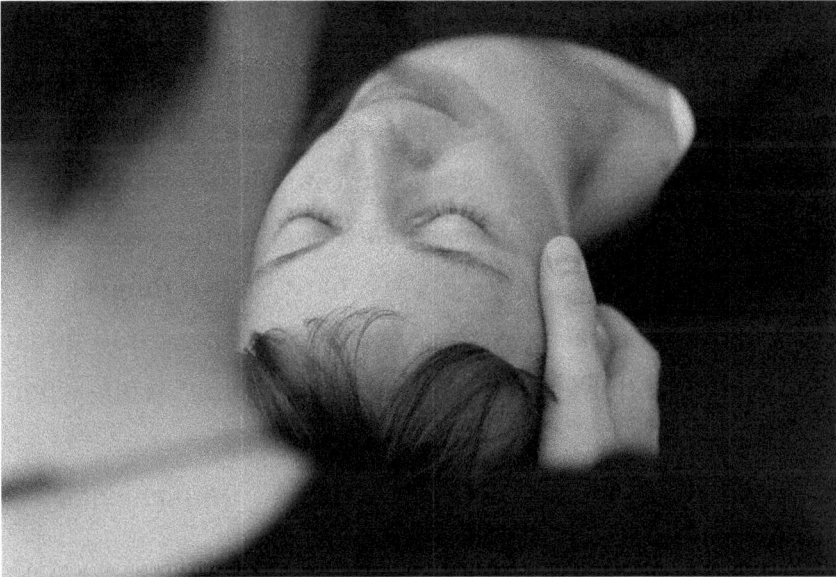

There are many different methods of holistic healing and every approach is personalized. Wellness means different things to different people depending on their personality, environment and biological make-up. As you study on the different holistic approaches to determine which best suits your health concerns, the common idea is that wellness needs to be addressed as a whole.

According to Thomas Edison, "The doctor of the future will give no medicine, but will interest patients in the maintenance of the human frame, in diet, and in the prevention of disease."

While many holistic healing methods may seem strange, the practice is slowly becoming a popular alternative in many countries and cultures. This chapter will discuss the most popular holistic healing approaches that have made their way into the mainstream health and wellness sector. The field of scientific medicine is so broad and even complementary, natural or alternative therapies cannot be clearly defined in its diversity. To put things in perspective, natural therapies are used in place of traditional medicine are often called "alternative medicine" while when holistic approaches are used in conjunction with conventional medical practices are called "complementary medicine."

This chapter will discuss different holistic therapies, uses and benefits that have changed the way many people across the globe manage medical care. It is important to note that with holistic healing, the body is also considered as an energy biofield, commonly known as aura. Do not be spooked out when you read about holistic therapies and the theories behind it. It is ancient wisdom but science has been catching up on this fact.

Did you know for a fact that body cells emanate light of about one inch outside the skin? Science says that this is how cells communicate. One's energy system is affected or influenced by what you do to your body, how you take care of it, how you think, and what you believe as well as your social interactions and environmental situations. Your holistic wellness is also interconnected with other people and life on the planet.

When you think about it, your own healing and wellness is essential to others' healing and well-being, too. As you read about different holistic methods, have an open mind so you can really look inside yourself and identify which approaches can help bring balance to your unique health needs.

1. Acupressure

In one of the previous chapters, acupuncture was mentioned. Acupuncture, as contrasted to acupressure, involves needles. But the concept is the same. Acupressure practitioners will apply force to specific pressure points in the body using their fingers, elbows, hands or feet. The points are referred to as "meridians." The leading belief behind this method is that the body contains life energy or *ch'i* and this energy is carried through the meridian channels. When the meridians are obstructed due to imbalance, illnesses can happen. When pressure is applied to the blocked meridians, the *ch'i* can flow freely once more and will restore health and wellness. While research is still ongoing regarding the truth of this theory, many studies have proven that positive results have been brought by acupressure. Some of the most common benefits that people get from the practice of acupressure is reduced anxiety, relief from migraine and even decreased nausea for patients who undergo chemotherapy.

2. *Aromatherapy*

There has been a growing trend on the use of essential oils to foster health and healing. This holistic approach is called aromatherapy. Simply put, it addresses the need for balance through one's physical senses. Essential oils are oils that are extracted from seeds, flowers, leaves, or roots of plants and concentrated. The concentrated oils can then be used through inhalation infusion and in some cases, ingestion. Others mix essential oils into rubs that can be massaged into one's skin. People use aromatherapy to:

- stimulate relaxation

- cure inflammation

- decrease feeling of physical pain

- reduce anxiety

3. Hydrotherapy

Up to 60% of the human body is composed of water so it is very likely that an imbalance can be treated by water. This is the concept of hydrotherapy or *balneotherapy*. Water is utilized for therapeutic purposes. Balneotherapy has been used since 1700 BC. Hydrotherapy is not just about drinking water, though. Hydration can be done through douches, wraps and mudpacks. It is believed that water can improve and treat skin conditions such as acne, swelling and breakouts as well as help relieve anxiety and boost immune systems.

4. Ayuverda

Ayuverdic medicine began in India and has been practiced for many centuries. Ayuverda promotes inclusive and total wellness through the use of herbs, special diets, and massage therapy to bring balance to the spirit, mind and body. The word "ayuverda" comes from the Sanskrit *ayur* and *veda* which means the "science of life" or "life built on knowledge".

The objective of Ayuverda is to halp people have a balanced life so that they can live long and healthy. It opposes the use of prescription medicine and complex surgeries as well as the idea of prolonged suffering. Ayuverdic medicine is one of the oldest methods in the world and even though there is written records now, most of the practices have been handed down from generations to generations through word of mouth.

Ayuverdic medicine can be combined with yoga and meditation. The use of herbs and accompanying practices have been said to help cure irritable bowel syndrome, chronic constipation, and chronic fatigue. It also helps reduce the risk of obesity, cure acne and minimize pain caused by some illnesses. One report on Ayuverdic medicine according to University of Maryland Medical Center notes that some autoimmune, digestive, hormonal and inflammatory conditions can be treated using Ayuverdic medicine to some benefits, including asthma, anxiety, dementia, high blood pressure, herpes, dysmenorrhea, PMS, Parkinsons' disease, Alzheimer's and even cancer.

According to Ayuverdic practice, there are six stages of illnesses:

Stage 1 – Accumulation

Stage 2 – Aggravation

Stage 3 – Dissemination

Stage 4 – Localization

Stage 5 – Manifestation

Stage 6 – Disruption

Ayuverda focuses on what you do on a daily basis so that you can prevent accumulating illnesses and in turn prevent the other stages from happening. In today's world, people are bombarded by stress which brings about sleep deprivation and can result in weak immune systems. When bad cells accumulate in the body, the situation can be aggravated as the immune system has no ability to fight them off. Disease can disseminate and localize in bodily organs and manifest as ailments or symptoms. Balance is disrupted. From stress alone, people can suffer from heart diseases, breathing dysfunctions, blood pressure problems and other nervous system illnesses. Preventative wellness is very, very important.

Regarding safety precautions, though, it should be noted that Ayurvedic medicine utilizes many different products and practices. As with any treatment, it is best to proceed with caution and never to use an approach without the direction and supervision of a trained professional. For instance, there are some herbs that cannot be combined with traditional medicines. Also, ingesting some metals and minerals can be poisonous. And while it is a popular, age-tested practice in India and other parts of Asia, there are not enough clinical trials in the Western medical community to support its effectivity and benefits.

5. Biofeedback

Body functions can be voluntary or involuntary. Voluntary actions include raising your hand, closing your eyes, opening your mouth, taking a step, etc. Involuntary functions include breathing, blood pressure, heart rate and other functions that are controlled by the nervous system. You don't do these things consciously, you don't think about them, but they happen as a response to what is happening around you. For example, when you are anxious, excited or scared, your heart will beat faster. Now, since these functions are controlled by your nervous system, you may think that you have no control over it—but you can influence it through biofeedback techniques.

Biofeedback is a holistic approach that will let you control your bodily processes. You can influence muscle tension, skin temperature, blood pressure and heart rate to address ailments such as headaches, persistent pain, migraine, incontinence, high blood pressure. A biofeedback therapist will work with a patient to determine bodily states and make a plan that includes exercises and relaxation techniques.

In initial biofeedback sessions, bodily functions will be measured using finger sensors or electrodes that are attached to the skin. The sensors will transmit a signal to an attached monitor and show an image that will represent a function that is not balanced (breathing, heart rate, muscle activity, etc.) The body's responses to stress are shown as they happen. When these are identified, a person will recognize what relaxation technique or exercise to apply in order to bring back balance.

This is the reason why biofeedback sessions are performed in a therapist's office where the devices are located. But after some time, the patient learns techniques to identify the rate of involuntary body functions, and he will know how to implement appropriate exercises and relaxation methods that will normalize said functions.

Easing up or relaxing reduces stress which aggravates the bodily functions and results in imbalance. The concept of biofeedback is that a person can harness mind over body power. It helps you fine tune your control over your body's involuntary functions. When you are aware of what is happening inside your body, you can do something to control it and make it better. For instance, you can do relaxation techniques when you feel that a headache is starting to stop the imbalance in your brain waves. Here are some relaxation techniques used in this holistic approach:

- Deep breathing

- Guided imagery – this is a technique where a person will concentrate on a definite image so that the mind can settle on this particular thing to bring relaxation.

- Mindfulness meditation – a popular method, this allows a person to be mindful and focus on his thoughts and disregard other negative feelings and thoughts that surround him. It brings calmness and promotes balance.

- Progressive muscle relaxation – this involves the constricting and releasing of particular muscle groups to bring relaxation.

6. Chiropractic

Do you deal with chronic joint pain, headaches, and backaches? Then chiropractic therapy may be what you need. It is more of a complementary rather than alternative therapy and is a widely acknowledge practice in the medical field. This holistic practice involves addressing nervous and musculoskeletal disorders. The concept is to restore mobility to one's arms, legs, neck, head, back and joints by applying force. People have joint pains as a result of injury in the tissues, hence there is restricted movement. The injury can be cause by poor posture, repetitive stress, or trauma caused by an event such as wrong lifting of weights.

Chiropractic procedures help adjust the affected area so that the patient's muscles and joints are loosened and they can be mobile again. When muscles and joints are loosened, the tissues around the joints start to heal, the inflammation subsides and pain is resolved. A lot of people have benefitted from this holistic, drug-free, non-invasive care. Chiropractic benefits include naturally improving:

- headaches

- back pain

- regular bowel movement

- focus, concentration and mental clarity

- neck pain

- joint pain

- ear infections

- arthritis

- asthma

- scoliosis

- organ functions

- blood pressures

7. Homeopathy

Have you heard of treating like with like? That is how homeopathy works. As with vaccines, the same substance that triggers hostile bodily reactions (when taken in large amounts) is used in smaller doses as a means to deal with the same symptoms. Homeopathy is not simple and using this holistic approach requires practitioners to collect all-encompassing information about their patients before they can recommend the right substance as a solution. This substance can be in tablet or liquid form and is highly diluted. The intake of the diluted substance wills kick-start the healing of the body's natural healing powers.

8. Naturopathy

Naturopathic medicine is a science-based approach to restore physical, psychological and biological balance using natural therapies. The principles behind naturopathy include the following:

- There is healing power in nature, meaning the body can heal itself and restore balance when the hindrances are removed.

- The cause, instead of the symptoms, should be identified and treated. The symptoms are only a manifestation of the imbalance that is happening on the inside. Naturopathy goes deeper than managing symptoms.

- It is important to do no harm. Naturopathy exerts a conscious effort to use non-invasive, gentle methods that will not cause any side effects.

- The doctor is regarded as a teacher. Naturopathic physicians or therapists should educate and empower their patients so that they can be responsible for their health, healing and lifestyle.

Naturopathy incorporates a wide range of treatments such as behavioral modification, acupuncture, homeopathy, herbal medicine, aromatherapy, and nutrition therapy.

9. Reflexology

More than a massage, reflexology targets specific areas of the body like the ears, feet and hands. It is believed that there are pressure points in these body parts that correspond to various bodily organs and systems and when pressed can bring a positive effect to respective organs and improve overall wellness.

Reflexology can be performed by the patient himself or it can be done by a trained reflexologist. This kind of holistic therapy has been used to accompany traditional treatments used to address anxiety, asthma, kidney problems, bladder issues, cancer and even diabetes. According to some studies, reflexology is proven to help decrease fatigue, improve sleep and enhance respiratory functions.

10. Reiki

This Japanese method that promotes relaxation is based on the idea that the reason we are alive is that a life force energy flows within us. It is believed that when this energy flow is weak, then we become unhealthy and when this energy flow is high, we can be healthy and happy. It is like spiritual healing—the practitioner will place his hands on a person's body as a means to eliminate negative energy or any blockages that cause the patient to feel weak. This channeled energy encourages emotional, physical, and mental healing. Practitioners and recipients of *reiki* believe of it as a manifestation of love, force and light. It is not a religion but it is believed to raise of spiritual levels, a holistic healing method that has a positive effect on spirit, soul and body.

Side Effects of Holistic Healing

One of the best advantages of holistic healing is that it has very minimal side effects. As long as the methods are used correctly, guidelines are followed and a reputable practitioner is selected to assist you in your holistic journey, then you do not have to worry. The worst that can happen is that you will have a lifestyle overhaul-your body will experience change, toxins will be eliminated as your body detoxifies, your mind will be free from stress, your emotions will be managed, you will have fresh and sufficient nutrients, and you will attain spiritual balance.

One thing that can be considered as a "side effect" is a healing crisis. It is a term used in the alternative medicine lingo to refer to a condition of the body wherein toxins that are being eliminated are poured into the bloodstream simultaneously, causing the body to experience a toxic overload until such time that everything is flushed out and the backlog is cleared. A person undergoing a healing crisis may suffer from headaches, nausea, and sensitivities to light and noise.

A healthy person with healing crisis is advised to lie down and rest in a dark and quiet room and drink herbal tea. For a person suffering from serious sickness like cancer, diabetes, arthritis or similar conditions, healing crisis may cause more than overload of stimulations and a qualified practitioner or therapist should assist them during the detoxification process.

While some traditional medical practitioners may view holistic healing with skepticism and reservation, there is presently a general acceptance for the positive impact and role that this alternative medicine plays in the health and wellness of patients that experience a variety of complaints.

Chapter Six: Holistic Healing in Action

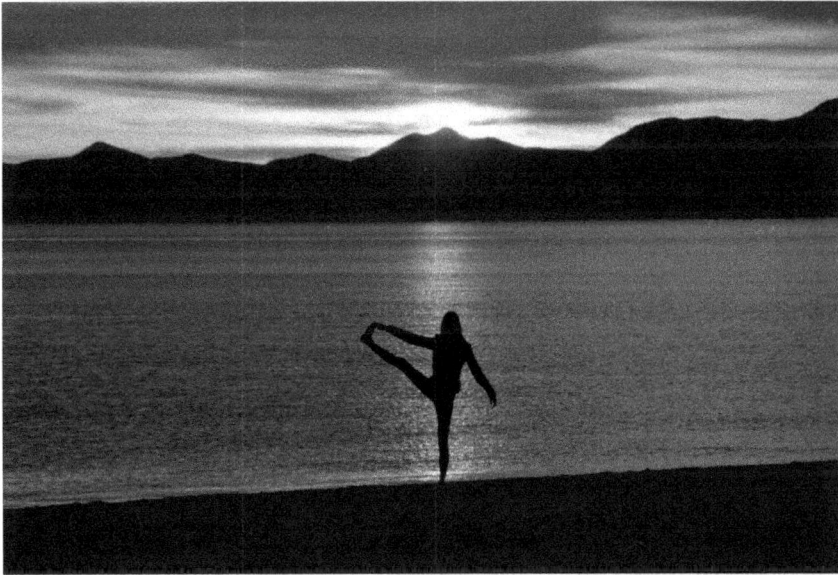

Healing is by no means static—it is a process that is constantly in motion. Healing your life is an exciting journey and an electrifying adventure you must take—do it!

In this chapter you will see how holistic healing helps manage common ailments and symptoms that people suffer. It is important to remember that when your health problem is severe, you should seek professional help. Holistic practitioners can help you identify the problem and design a suitable plan of treatment for you. (The examples mentioned in this chapter are common ailments that affect people. Included are simple yet effective means on how you can, on your own, take control of your health if you are facing said health challenges. It is not a single formula for success as every individual has unique needs.)

Managing Depression

Every person goes through life's ups and downs. Depression has been a prevalent mental illness that has plagued people from all ages, race, cultures and walks of life. Depression can be caused by significant loneliness, stressful events, challenges and change. Not everyone can bounce back easily from these situations and individuals can suffer prolonged bouts of sadness, emptiness, and isolation. Depressed people show symptoms of frustration, irritability, and apathy. They lose interest in normal activities that used to bring the pleasure. They have sleeping problems, low energy levels and poor appetite. Depression causes them to think of suicide or death. Not everyone can be easily diagnosed with depression as there are many levels and forms of this mental condition.

However, you don't have to be exhibiting these symptoms daily for 14 consecutive days in order for you to seek help. You have the choice and the power to stop this downward spiral before it gets worse. You can address it holistically and naturally.

Here is an example of a holistic assessment when it comes to addressing depression:

- Stressful situations can cause you to feel down and depressed.

- When your physical body is weak due to lack of sleep or poor nutrition, you will find it hard to face challenges of life with strength and positivity.

- When you are spiritually disconnected, your soul is frail and you cannot make positive choices. Hence, you suffer mentally and emotionally.

- When there is an imbalance in the financial, social and environmental factors of your life, it is not hard for you to become depressed.

You see, the condition (depression) should be viewed as a holistic concern and not as a problem of one part of your life. Everything is interconnected; when you understand that you can bring healing and health to the whole person as well. Here are three simple, natural steps you can take to manage depression and eventually bring back balance to your life or your loved ones who are suffering from it.

Change your diet.

You need to know that when you take in foods that have high sugar and simple carbohydrates (white rice, white cereal, white bread, pastries, sweets, refined sugars), you can experience abnormal levels of blood sugar. A significant spike or drop in levels will cause you to experience low energy, mood swings and aggravated depressive symptoms.

Stock up on Vitamin B.

B Vitamins (B1, B2, B6, B12) is important in maintaining a good level of energy in your body as well as your temper. These vitamins help synthesize neurotransmitters with help regulate hormones that control moods. Get vitamin B naturally from green leafy vegetables, avocados bananas and sunflower seeds. You can consult with a doctor if you need to take additional Vitamin B supplements as well.

Get acupuncture therapy.

Instead of antidepressant medicines, go for acupuncture. Studies have shown that people suffering from depression that were treated for 6 weeks with acupuncture showed significant improvements. You may need more than one acupuncture session, and make sure that you go to a licensed and trusted practitioner. However, for severe cases of depression, a different kind of treatment may be necessary.

Note: Depression and symptoms of depression is *not* a normal part of life. When it is affecting the quality of your life and your relationships, it is best to seek professional help for a detailed diagnosis and proper treatment options.

Beating Back Pains

Millions of people suffer from back pain. It is such a common problem all over the world. However, 95% of back pain cases do not require invasive procedures. The problem comes as people age or because of their posture, work or lifestyle. Bone strength and muscle elasticity are also factors that come into play.

Back pain should be treated not as a simple physical ailment. Some problems are not just caused by age or physical conditions. Oftentimes, people who are stressed suffer from back pains because stress causes toxins to be released into the body causing muscle spasms and tension. Poor nutrition can also cause degradation of bone density which can lead to back problems. Worrying, feeling bitter or harboring pain can also manifest in muscle pains. Again, holistic healing can help beat back pains.

Do yoga.

Various poses can cause your back muscles to stretch and relax (child's pose, downward dog, cat and camel, pigeon pose). Stretching and relaxing helps reduce the compression that builds up in your lower spine which in turn causes pain.

Shed off those excess pounds.

More weight means more pressure on your lower spine which causes muscle tension. You are also at risk to suffer from compression of nerves, disc bulges and spine injury.

Use herbal medicine.

Natural creams such as capsaicin can help you manage pain. The body transmits substance P when it is in pain, and the pain impulses in your brain is triggered causing an imbalance physically, mentally and emotionally.

When you use capsaicin (found in chili peppers), you reduce the amount of this neurotransmitter thereby reducing the pain levels. The cream is applied topically on the affected area and provides relief from pain.

Exercise properly.

First of all, you cannot simply stay in bed when your back is acting up. You need to move. Movement and exercise can actually address the pain and help your muscles heal faster. Secondly, you can't just make any movement. You have to know the right kind and amount of exercise that will properly address the problem. Usually low impact exercises done with moderate intensity will work well for back pains. You cannot squat or jump too much.

Try acupuncture.

The proper use of needles at specific "acupoints" will help trigger the transmission of pain-reducing hormones in your body. Acupuncture has been known to successfully treat chronic back pain.

Fight Chronic Fatigue

According to the Center for Disease Control (CDC), chronic fatigue syndrome is very prevalent. It is not a physical condition, but a mental one. People with chronic fatigue syndrome feels extremely worn out after exerting physical or mental effort, no matter how small. Sometimes, even brushing one's teeth can prove to be a gruesome task. Prescription medicines are not the only answer; you can try holistic healing through the following:

Nutrition therapy – ribose and vitamin D

Ribose is a vital sugar that the body needs to produce energy. Don't think table sugar and decide that you should eat more cookies! On the contrary, do not take in too much sugar like that or you will experience drops in your energy levels and eventually develop diabetes. You can take ribose supplements to reduce fatigue symptoms such as pain, mental haze and sleeping problems. Additionally, you need 1,000 to 4,000 IU of Vitamin D daily when you suffer from chronic fatigue.

Get enough sleep.

When you get ample sleep, the body is restored and energies are replenished. Healing processes take place during shuteye. When you get 8 hours of sleep every single night, you will find yourself more energized, strengthened and refreshed.

Graded exercise therapy.

Exercise does wonders for the body. Graded exercise involves stretching and guided motions that one can do on a daily basis to help the body gain energy and strength. As it is continued, the length and intensity can be increased to suit the requirements of a patient.

As with depression, living with chronic fatigue can be frustrating and overwhelming but that should not discourage you. You can take control of your life and feel better!

Managing Irritable Bowel Syndrome

A lot of people suffer from chronic bouts of diarrhea/constipation, abdominal pain, bloating, and cramping. These symptoms are caused by the gastrointestinal disorder called IBS or irritable bowel syndrome. Millions of people are affected and even though there is no specific cause attributed to this illness, it is widely believed that stress is a contributing factor. There is also an abnormality in the communication of the gut and the brain therefore the imbalance in the digestive system. While you may not suffer any long-term damage from IBS, everyday life can be miserable. Here are some holistic approaches you can apply to help you manage IBS symptoms:

Yoga and meditation.

As mentioned earlier, stress is a contributing factor to this ailment that plagues millions. It can increase the frequency of the symptoms and make them worse. By doing yoga and meditation practices, you can help manage or reduce stress levels.

Use of essential oils.

Peppermint can help ease the symptoms of IBS including abdominal pains, cramping and bloating. Peppermint can also pacify distention and gas. You can take peppermint tea or peppermint oil capsules.

Fiber and probiotics intake.

The body needs fiber as it can improve the regularity of the stool. It will also alleviate cramping and bloating. Probiotics, on the other hand, reduces abdominal pain. People with IBS do not have a healthy gut flora and need probiotic organisms to maintain a balance in their digestive tract.

Taking a Holistic Holiday

There are many daily issues of life that causes symptoms and ailments that can be addressed by taking a holistic holiday. Everyone needs to take a break every so often, but holistic holidays don't mean having a 'staycation' or lazing around the pool. Just journeying far from home to put the stress behind you won't work—you may get a respite from it while you are away, but when you come back, the issues of everyday life will still be there and you will encounter the same stressors and strains. Holistic holidays mean that you do something to gain long-term benefits and balance for your body, soul and spirit.

With holistic holidays, your goal is to reconnect with yourself, find purpose, relieve stress and strengthen one's physical well-being. Holistic holidays involve therapy to improve general health and restore spiritual, emotional and mental balance. Like holistic healing approaches holistic holidays are unique to every individual and focus on the whole self. Take one today and get your life back!

Chapter Seven: Holistic Healing for Emotional and Psychological Problems

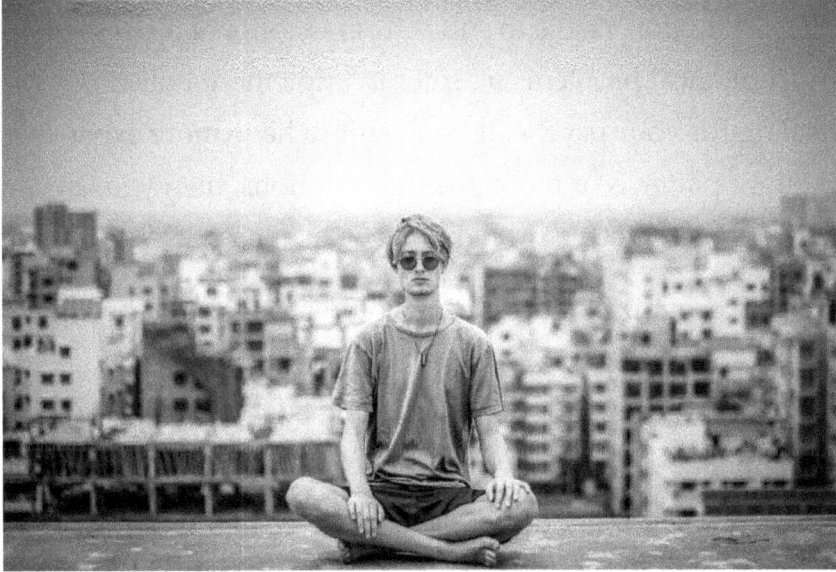

Emotional wellness is not just a simple state of being happy or being free from stress. Being emotionally healthy means you can recognize, assess and impart your feelings with other people. It means you can navigate through your emotions and manage your responses or reactions.

Holistic healing for emotional and mental issues requires a restoration of balance and wellness in your inner self, our consciousness. Holistic healing for mental problems does not necessarily equate to directly treating a mental condition—but mental wellness means that one is empowered to improve his thinking patterns using complementary, natural methods. It means negativity is blocked and positivity takes root.

You don't have to suffer from emotional distress or psychological problems in order to implement holistic healing for your psyche. If you want to have more expansive thought patterns or more positive emotions, then you can address these needs through holistic healing.

Recognize that restoring your emotions and healing your mind is closely interconnected. Your thoughts, your feelings, your emotions and what you believe are in a continual dance with each other. You can't address one without considering the other. Your beliefs guide your feelings, and your emotions can affect your thoughts.

Holistic healing for your emotions and your mind go hand in hand. For example, when you decide to impute more positivity on how you view and talk about yourself, your emotions will also shift in a constructive manner. As you recognize and validate your feelings, you will discover that emotions such as anger or fear will find no place in your heart or mind.

Understanding Emotions and Mindsets

There are a variety of emotions and different shades
to it. Being aware of your emotions is the initial step to
holistic healing leading to positive feelings and thoughts.
Feeling all kinds of emotions is healthy. From joy, anger,
fear, sadness, disgust, or nervousness—all emotions,
positive or negative should be acknowledged. Emotions let
you know how you are interpreting what happens in you
and around you. Emotions are energetic indicators and
responses to the subliminal inner talk that goes on in your
mind. Feeling emotions, regardless of their intensity, can
help you understand what is going on inside of you and
help you identify where you need healing and wholeness.
Here are some areas that can be addressed:

Addressing inner talk

The inner voice is very powerful—it can make or
break you. It can cause you to be happy or lonely, a success
or a failure, healthy or sick. It is normal for people to have
more negative thoughts than positive ones and to apply
holistic healing means that you recognize these thoughts as
helpful indicators of what needs to stay and what needs to

go away. What are the things that need to go away?
Negative self-talk, negative mindset patterns, and stinking
thinking. While negative thinking may have some positive
advantages, it is best to start your holistic healing journey
with positivity through improving your self-talk and the
way you think about yourself.

Healing damaged emotions

Negative mindset patterns can be caused by past
experiences and traumas. These lead to damaged emotions
and unhealthy beliefs that limit your potential. When
negative emotions interfere with the quality of your life and
cause you to act in detrimental ways, then you know that
you are imbalanced. In order to heal, you need to release
past pains and the emotions that are tied to it.

Shifting in the moment

You can practice to shift your emotions in the
moment—from negative to positive. For example, someone
says something bad to you, anger or hurt will rise up. You
can counter this with a positive emotion: do not react. When
you practice this regularly, you will also see an
improvement in your overall mental health. It is not easy in

the beginning but with continued practice, you will teach your mind the value of choosing the right emotion that is most beneficial to your health in the moment.

Anger management

Feeling angry is normal. It is a healthy and natural response given specific situations. It only becomes detrimental to your holistic health when you leave it unchecked. Anger can cause so much negativity in your mind, soul and body. It can also cause havoc on other people's lives and in your relationships. Anger is a very powerful emotion that you need to rein in and use to your benefit.

Your mind, will and emotions are connected intimately to your physical body and there is a reciprocal effect. For example, nervousness, anxiety or excitement can cause you to feel as if you have a pit in your stomach or as if there are fluttering butterflies in it. There can be a physical manifestation of emotions and thoughts. Suffice it to say, negative emotions, trash in your thoughts and restrictive beliefs can result in disruption in your body resulting in physical illness. When you are sick, you lose the opportunity to live a good quality life.

Conversely, positive feelings, positive thoughts and positive belief systems can bring about a spontaneous physical healing even with no medical involvement. That is why they say laughter is the best medicine. A proverb says that laughter and joy brings healing to the bones. Positivity can correct imbalances in all aspects of health.

When you address emotional and mental well-being, you will find that the positive change will also be evident in other elements of health in your life. With the physical aspect, you will notice that you are more confident, you will have better posture as you carry yourself taller, and you will be more relaxed. Your spiritual health will also improve when you let go of negative emotions and connect with the divine. Your social relations will pick up as you have a more positive outlook in life. Many health issues may be resolved when you address emotional and psychological wholeness.

Now, even if you are in good physical health, it is also important to attend to emotional and mental healing. And if you already have good health in those three areas, then work on the rest. Having inner peace, happiness, acceptance and self-love will work wonders in your life and in your relationships.

Chapter Eight: Holistic Healing for Everyday Life

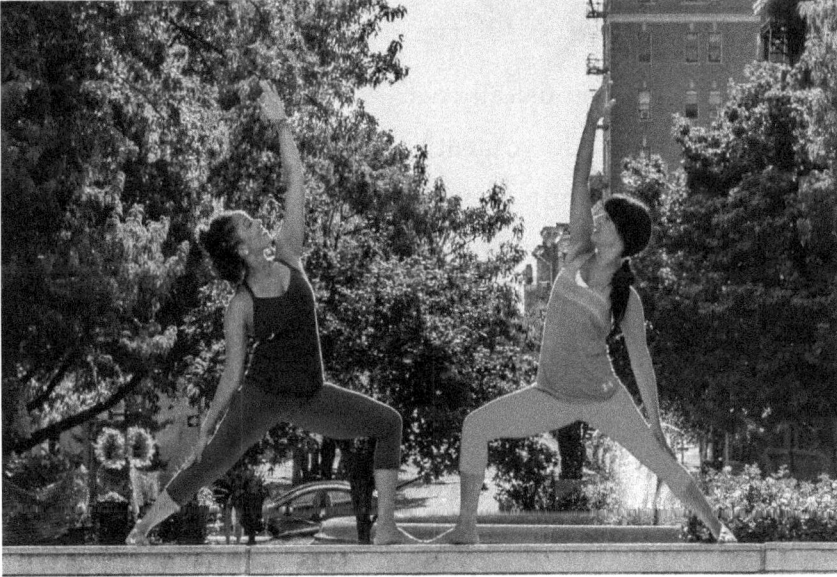

It is said that you are the sum of your daily habits; what you do repeatedly, regularly, can define you. This means that you can improve your holistic health on a daily basis. Every day, there is something that you do, say, think or feel that either contributes or takes away from your holistic health. Think about these questions as they pertain to factors that affect holistic health:

PHYSICAL

Nutrition

- What do you usually eat?
- How much do you eat?
- How frequently do you eat?
- Do you eat only what you like?
- Is your diet nutrition-based?
- What is your guiding principle: live to eat or eat to live?

Exercise

- What kinds of exercise or physical activity do you do?
- How often do you exercise?
- How long do you exercise?
- Do you have strength to do your daily tasks?

Physical Image

- Are you happy with how you look?
- Do you want to change your weight?

MENTAL

Mindsets

- Are you a positive thinker?
- Do you focus on the good that happens or the bad?
- Are you grateful for what you have?
- Do you worry about the things that you don't have?
- Are you anxious about tomorrow (future)?

Goal Setting

- Do you set smart goals?
- Do you work toward your goals?
- Do you get distracted by trivial things in the pursuit of your goals?
- Do you set a time-frame in achieving your goals?
- Do you periodically assess where you are in life?
- Do you know why you are going where you are going (direction in life)?

INNER TALK

- Do you talk to yourself?
- What kind of voice do you use with yourself?
- Do you get angry with yourself when something goes wrong?
- What do you think of yourself?
- How do you feel when you look at yourself in a mirror?
- Do you compliment yourself?
- What do you tell yourself when other compliment you?
- How do you feel and what do you tell yourself when someone criticizes you?

SPIRITUALITY

- Do you know your purpose in life?
- Are you aware of your divine connection?
- Do you live life with direction or just wing it as it comes?
- Does everything you do bring meaning and fulfillment to you?

OUTLOOK IN LIFE

- How do you see life in general?
- Do you like solving problems or complaining about them?
- Do you have control over your life or other people and situations control you?
- Are you a spectator or participator?

VIEW ON HEALTH

- Do you accept responsibility for your health?
- Do you do what feels good or you do what is right?
- Do you understand how your body works?
- Do you leave taking care of your health to doctors?

OUTLLOK PERTAINING TO OTHER PEOPLE

- How do you see other people?
- Do you judge people and generalize them into categories such as good, bad, ugly, lazy, suspicious, trustworthy, or mixtures of different characteristics?
- How does your perception of other people influence the way you treat them?

HANDLING INFORMATION and TIME

- Do you seek answers and ask questions in order to get information?
- Do you lounge around and idly sit in front of the television and waste time because you don't like the life you have right now?
- Is your free time spent productively or with just entertaining yourself?
- Do you set aside time to discover more about yourself and improve?
- Do you understand how your physical health is affected by your mindsets, belief systems, emotions, skills, work, environment, and social interactions?

FORMS OF ENTERTAINMENT/ENJOYMENT

- What television shows do you usually watch?
- Are you always on social media?
- What kinds of music do you listen to?
- Do you read books?
- Do you study to gain information so you can improve your life?

STRESS MANAGEMENT

- What is your initial reaction during stressful situations?
- Do you immediately push away negative thoughts?
- Do you know how to handle anger and mood swings?
- Do you know that mental and emotional stress can affect your physical body? What do you do about it?

Getting the honest answers to these questions will give you an idea about how you view your holistic health, how you think about it and what you usually do about it. If you see that your answers do not help you sustain holistic health, then you need to apply certain changes that will improve your holistic health.

5 Simple Steps to Holistic Healing Every Day

Simple steps, when incorporated in your everyday life can bring a positive change and inspire quality living. You don't need to memorize and implement 25 or a hundred things in order to gain holistic health especially when you have a very busy daily schedule, so this chapter narrows it down to five (yes, just 5!) simple steps to bring balance and health back into your life.

The fundamental principle of these five steps is mindfulness. To enhance your holistic health will require more than simply eating well and exercising often. Besides, you cannot force yourself to eat and exercise when your mind is not into it. The mind is one of the first things you need to focus on if you want to begin a journey towards holistic wellness.

Do outdoor yoga.

While indoor yoga, at home or in a gym, is also beneficial, take the time to go outdoors. You need the fresh air and natural environment to help your body relax and be in tune with your inner self, your spirit, your center. If you have children, going outdoors will benefit them, too. They can join you for yoga, or they can play and enjoy nature while you focus on your poses.

Not only can you find your center and relax, you can also have guided meditation and say affirmations while you are doing yoga.

Start mindfulness in the morning.

Mornings mean you have a fresh new day ahead of you. Before the stress of life creeps in and you have to handle frustrations and anxiety, make sure to set aside time every morning to be alone and practice mindfulness. This will help set you up for emotional and mental balance; you will have a peaceful mindset that will empower you to take on whatever life throws your way.

Eliminate toxicity.

Many things cause stress. It is different for everyone—it can come from food, products, other people, situations, or your environment. If you want to improve your holistic health, you must learn to identify the stressors in your life and remove them. Here are some tips on how you can help remove stress or toxicity from your daily life:

- **Declutter your office table, your bedroom drawers or your kitchen counters.**

  A decluttered space will aid in decluttering your mind. At work, take some time to tidy up your table or cubicle. At home, do the same thing. Now you don't have to declutter your whole home all at once, that alone may cause you undue stress. But take it one cabinet at a time, one room at a time. Soon enough, you will have removed all the clutter that you didn't know causes you undue stress every time you are around or in the midst of it.

- **Try deep breathing exercise.**
  Breathe in fresh air to energize you and breathe out all those toxins from your body.

- **Place a vase of flowers in the house or in your office table.**

  Sometimes, seeing something beautiful from nature helps you flush out toxicity. Moreover, it is a reminder for you to take a break, "stop and smell the roses."

- **Throw away (or delete) items that bring up bad memories.**
  Do you still have that picture of your old flame on your phone? That rejection letter in your drawer? When things you have in your possession don't help

build you up and only cause you to remember pain and hurtful thoughts, then it is time to let them go.

Practice mindful eating.

Yes, you should eat healthy and get proper nutrition. Mindful eating goes beyond that. It means that you enjoy eating and take the stress out of it. It is important to have an awareness of what you are eating and why you are eating it. It is also good to attune yourself to bodily cues such as hunger, tiredness or feeling stressed so that you know when it is time to eat because your body needs it and not just because you are stressed out, giving in to cravings or turning to food for comfort.

Here is good advice: choose to eat at the dining table and not in front of the television so you can focus on what you are eating and your mindset towards eating. Edward Stanley wisely said, "Those who think they have no time for healthy eating…will sooner or later have to find time for illness."

Practice affirmations.

It is not easy to control your thoughts, especially if you have experienced trauma or a negative background that often gives way to negative thoughts and feelings. Holistic healing, through affirmations, will allow you to input specific positive contemplations that will inspire you to create a more positive and beneficial mindset. Here are some affirmations that you can tell yourself every single day:

- I respect my body. It is mine and I make right choices for it.

- My body is my responsibility—I take care of it.

- I think peaceful and gentle thoughts.

- I accept myself.

- I believe in myself.

- My emotions are healthy.

- I am true to myself.

- I forgive myself.

- I forgive others, I love, I let go of negativity and hurt.

- I learn from my mistakes.

- Life is good, I will live today to the fullest.

- I have confidence in myself.

- I can do anything I set my mind to.

- I eat properly, rest well and exercise regularly to enjoy optimal health.

- I never give up.

When you practice daily, inspiring affirmations, you are effectively bringing positivity, encouragement, and motivation in your life.

These are simple things you can do every day without much effort. But as you consistently are mindful of it, you are developing good habits that lead to holistic healing and optimal health. Don't despise the day of small beginnings. Start with five and soon you will find yourself committed to good "whole self" health practices.

Chapter Nine: Why People Use Holistic Healing Practices

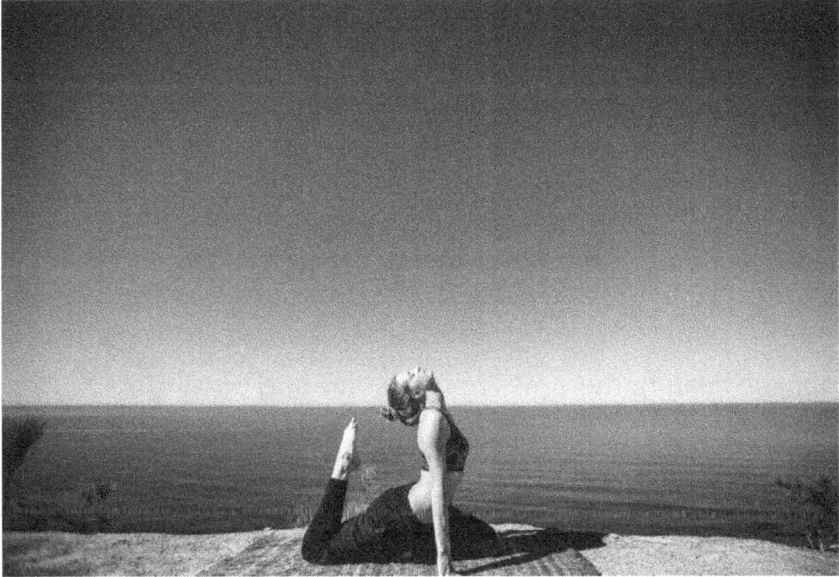

Peter Shepherd said, "Healing comes from taking responsibility: to realize that it is you – and no one else – that creates your thoughts, your feelings and your actions." Holistic healing stresses the value of you taking control over your life to create balance, harmony and wellness. This is one of the reasons holistic health and healing has gained popularity over the years.

Complementary Holistic Approaches

Holistic healing empowers people. Other reasons why people turn to alternative or complementary holistic approaches are the following:

Holistic healing therapies make one feel better

People who suffer from ailments such as cancer use holistic healing therapies to find some sort of comfort during the time of their illness or medical treatments. While there is no known evidence that holistic therapies can cure or prevent cancer, it is widely accepted that such practices can help with certain symptoms associated with cancer and chemotherapy such as hot flushes and pain.

How is this important? How you feel towards your illness and the treatment you are undergoing plays a big part in how you cope and how you heal. Remember that a person should be treated as a whole and not just in parts. As holistic healing techniques focus on reducing stress and promoting relaxation, patients are able to manage their emotions, alleviate their fears and anxiety, and improve their sense of health and wellness.

Holistic healing practices can minimize symptoms or side effects.

Treatment for progressive ailments such as cancer can cause adverse side effects. Growing evidence shows that some holistic healing techniques can help control these side effects. For example, acupuncture can mitigate sick feelings caused by chemotherapy drugs or radiation. It can also help relive sores and pain when there is surgery.

Holistic healing practices give the patient a sense of purpose and control.

When medical doctors make decisions regarding your treatment plans, you often feel helpless and even scared. You are already unhealthy and yet you don't have control over what can happen to you. In contrast, holistic healing lets the patient take on an active role with regards to his treatment, recovery and healing, as he works with a therapist/practitioner. Taken in context with the principle of a "whole person", it does have positive effects on one's emotional and mental well-being which in turn can positively affect his physical health.

Holistic healing is natural.

Patients get fed up with so many aggressive procedures and medicines so they prefer holistic healing techniques. These are natural, non-toxic, and non-invasive.

Holistic healing offers comfort.

Holistic practitioners take the time to understand the patient as a "whole person". They spend time talking to gather information that will be enough to create a treatment plan. Patients who are suffering from medical conditions tend to get comfort and contentment from all these: touch, talk and time. The holistic practitioner can help improve the quality of the patient's life by being supportive throughout the treatment and making the patient feel cared for.

Holistic healing encourages the patient to stay positive.

People use holistic healing therapies so that they will feel hopeful about what they are going through and this positive vibe will help them cope through difficult times.

Holistic healing boosts the immune system.

Holism is about creating balance and positivity and when patients feel good, stress levels are reduced and their immune systems are strengthened. This is beneficial for cancer patients as well as people suffering from mental disorders because often, medical conditions are aggravated when the immune system is weak.

How Holistic Health and Healing should be practiced

Holistic healing focuses not just on treating the illness or preventing it, but on achieving a higher level of well-being. There are two sides to it: on one end are people trying out different approaches and methods that will improve their condition. A holistic practitioner will help them identify the best health principles to apply, the holistic medicine to be utilized as well as other factors that will be considered to support the natural healing powers of one's body. The whole condition and the whole person is considered so that it is not just about eliminating symptoms but addressing the real problem. The symptoms are only used as a guide to figure out which area needs attention.

On the other end are people who are healthy and yet are continually exploring daily practices that can propel them towards optimal health. This end of the health continuum exists because people are encouraged by the positive effects that a good quality life brings—energy, happiness, enthusiasm, and hope for a healthy future.

There is no doubt that a lot of people do care about their health and give their best efforts to maintain it. However, not everyone will address the whole pie, but just a portion. You will find individuals who have great eating, exercise and sleeping habits and yet neglect the care of their mental and emotional health by not allowing themselves to rest and relax. There are people who work with a passion, enjoy creativity and a sense of life's meaning and yet compromise their sleep and diet.

Do you see the dilemma here? People are not very adept at giving attention to the whole person so a part or two is sacrificed and suffers. You need to learn to pay attention to everything about you—in the midst of your busy life, you have to discover what you are forgetting to care for. Do your best to have a complete approach to meeting your health needs in every area of your life. The purpose of this book is for you to understand the importance of holistic health and healing and to apply it in your life.

Start Small, Start Today

Even though you are not suffering from a medical condition, you can create a self-care path that will take you on a journey to wellness. To develop this personal plan, you should categorize the parts that will be addressed and choose an activity that will benefit you in that aspect in a meaningful way.

To start with, choose only one activity. When you develop it into a healthy habit, you can add more activities to promote holistic health. Note that it should not be a difficult or extreme activity otherwise you will give up and lose your sense of balance.

Here is a sample personal plan you can check out and use as inspiration to create your own:

Element of Health	Activity	Check when done (/)
Physical	Brisk walk 10 minutes a day	
Physical	Hydrate, drink 10	

	glasses of water daily	
Physical	Sleep 8 hours	
Physical	Eat more vegetables and fruits	
Mental	15-minute daily meditation	
Mental	Read one inspirational book a week	
Emotional	Practice deep breathing to manage stress	
Emotional	Forgive someone	
Spiritual	Pray everyday	
Spiritual	Read a devotional	
Social	Connect with a friend once a week	
Social	Reach out and talk to someone you don't know	
Financial/Economic	Set aside a small amount for savings	

Financial/Economic	Invest	
Environmental	Avoid noise	
Environmental	Segregate	

Make your personal plan today!

Element of Health	Activity	Check when done (/)
Physical		
Mental		
Emotional		
Spiritual		
Social		
Financial/Economic		
Environmental		

Chapter Ten: Choosing a Holistic Provider

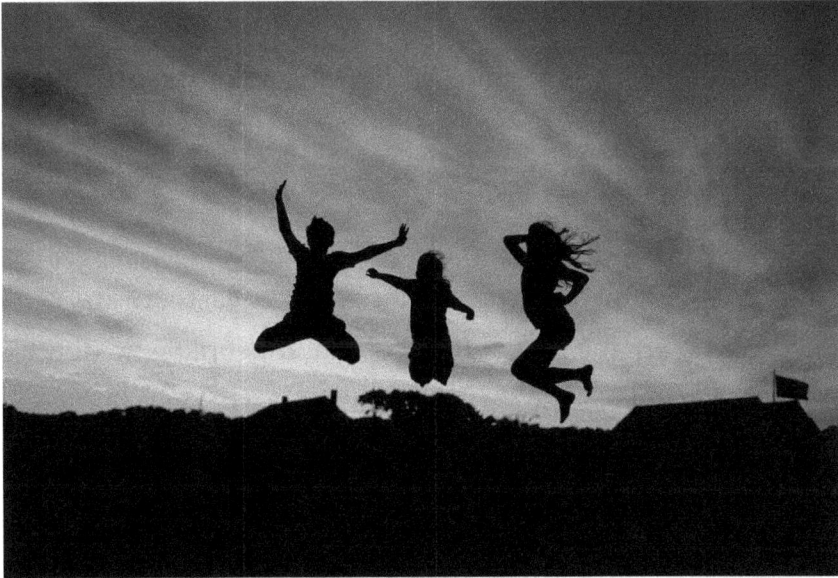

Again and again, it is important to stress that holistic healing is different for different people. What works well for others might not do so for you. Not everyone will want or will benefit from holistic treatments. When people are not comfortable with the approach, it will do them no good as there will be no balance. They will be better off staying with their medical practitioner. But if your heart and mind is set on achieving holistic healing, understand that you will experience best results when you take the time to find the holistic practitioner that is best suited to help you on your journey.

Tips in Choosing a Holistic Provider

Use the following as a guide in choosing a holistic provider:

Don't just go to anyone.

As with all other professional practices, there are people who are the best at their jobs, and people who don't do well. Do not choose the first holistic practitioner that you find. Get a second or even third opinion. Ask for recommendations from people you trust like a relative, friend or colleague, previous patients who have experienced significant health improvement, or from credible health organizations is your area.

Do your own research.

It is important to check the professional's background: education or training, specialization, experience, and affiliation with professional holistic organizations. What is this doctor's view and treatment philosophy? Do they mirror your own?

Consider how you feel about him/her.

Does this doctor make you feel comfortable? Does he/she respect your concerns and your views? Holistic healing is not one-sided. It is a team effort between the patient and the provider. If one is not comfortable with the other, there will be no harmony and they won't make any progress. Make sure that your holistic provider is someone that you will enjoy working with.

Check how much time he/she spends on your appointments.

Is he/she in a rush to talk about your concerns or does he/she allow you enough time to navigate through your issues and address needs? Choose someone whom you feel and see spends enough time to understand what you are going through and how best he/she can help you.

Does he/she ask the right questions?

Be prepared to answer tons of questions about your eating, sleeping and exercise habits, religious beliefs, relationships, environmental situations and more. This will help him/her gain understanding of you as a "whole" person.

Carefully consider the treatment options.

Does the wellness plan include other holistic approaches and not just prescription medicines? The holistic practitioner should have checked and considered lifestyle and medical factors hand in hand to determine what could contribute to your ailment and how to best deal with it.

Holistic doctors will educate their patients about the benefits of lifestyle change in order to achieve holistic healing and health. The doctor will offer different treatment plans that will empower and make the patient accountable for his own health. For example, the holistic practitioner may advise diet change such as removing processed food from one's diet and reducing calorie intake. He/she may advise the patient to undergo spiritual counseling or psychotherapy to address relational or mental health issues. Alternative therapies such as acupuncture, chiropractic care, naturopathy and the likes. It really depends on the assessment of individual medical conditions and all health elements factored in.

It is important to note that a holistic doctor will not suggest that you can heal a broken leg by taking some Asian herbal pill—that simply is not realistic. The wise and professional holistic practitioner knows when medication or surgery is needed and will not insist on natural or alternative approaches that may endanger the life of his patient. The best holistic practitioners will use everything that is available to help the patient heal and be healthy.

Conclusion

Hippocrates said, "The greatest medicine of all is to teach people not to need it." That is what holistic wholeness is all about.

Unfortunately, a lot of people tend to shy away from a holistic lifestyle or holistic healing methods because they are not certain what it entails. Simply put, it is living holistically—physically, mentally, emotionally, financially, socially, spiritually, environmentally—in the most natural way. It is an unpretentious way of understanding and caring for your whole self. It is so simple, yet many people forget about it because of the fast pace and stress of modern society.

Holistic health means that your body, soul and mind are linked and whatever happens to one part will eventually affect the others. Sicknesses, disease and disorders often come as a result of an imbalance. There are many approaches to holistic health and healing and each individual will discover a unique, personal methodology that will apply to them. It is all about balance and quality. It is all about you being responsible for your life. Take action so you can live life to the fullest.

Let me leave you with these thoughts: One, quality of life is unique to every person. You cannot compare your life with another person's. What is significant to you may be inconsequential to your brother or friend. Don't stress about it. Discover what will make YOU healthy and happy and work towards it. Two, your health is your responsibility and your blessing. You can achieve balance when you take charge of your life. When you discover something that fosters physical wellness and nurtures your soul, give it room in your life. Investing in yourself is not selfish at all–it is vital to your health. And when you are healthy, you have the power to achieve your dreams and live a happy, fulfilled life.

Photo Credits

Page Photo by user Ars Electronica via Flickr.com,

https://www.flickr.com/photos/arselectronica/4897601102/

Page Photo by user Tony Cecala via Flickr.com,

https://www.flickr.com/photos/tonycecala/29673141774/

Page Photo by user Ars Electronica via Flickr.com,

https://www.flickr.com/photos/arselectronica/4897600538/

Page Photo by user Ars Electronica via Flickr.com,

https://www.flickr.com/photos/arselectronica/4897006895/in/
photostream/Page Photo by user via Flickr.com,

Page Photo by user Ars Electronica via Flickr.com,

https://www.flickr.com/photos/arselectronica/4897007273/

Page Photo by user Hamza Butt via Flickr.com,

https://www.flickr.com/photos/149902454@N08/35545212845
/

Page Photo by user Francois D via Flickr.com,

https://www.flickr.com/photos/frfrdufour/15314472983/

References

"What Are Holistic Practices?" – University of Minnesota

https://www.takingcharge.csh.umn.edu/what-are-holistic-practices

"Principles of Holistic Medicine" – AHHA.org

https://ahha.org/selfhelp-articles/principles-of-holistic-medicine/

"What is Holistic Medicine" – WebMD.com

https://www.webmd.com/balance/guide/what-is-holistic-medicine#1

"What is Holistic Medicine" – My – Holistic – Healing.com

http://www.my-holistic-healing.com/what-is-holistic-healing.html

"4 Ways Holistic Health is Changing Traditional Medicine … And How You Can Benefit" – Medium.com

https://medium.com/thrive-global/4-ways-holistic-health-is-changing-traditional-medicine-and-how-you-can-benefit-e334e989041c

"Holistic Healing Therapies" - My – Holistic – Healing.com

http://www.my-holistic-healing.com/holistic-healing-therapies.html

"The Beginner's Guide to Alternative Medicine —and Exactly How It Works" – MyDomaine.com

https://www.mydomaine.com/holistic-healing-practices

"20 Mind-Body Treatments That Actually Work" – Prevention.com

https://www.prevention.com/life/a20434786/alternative-therapies-that-heal-health-problems/

"Integrative medicine: Alternative becomes mainstream" – Mayoclinic.org

https://www.mayoclinic.org/healthy-lifestyle/consumer-health/in-depth/alternative-medicine/art-20045267